# Your Family's Hunt for Wellness

A Guide to Finding the Best
Chiropractic Care for Life!

# Your Family's Hunt for Wellness

## A Guide to Finding the Best Chiropractic Care for Life!

By Estela Hunt, DC

ISBN: 978-1-945446-13-9

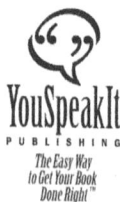

YouSpeakIt
PUBLISHING
The Easy Way
to Get Your Book
Done Right ™

www.YouSpeakItPublishing.com

# *Dedication*

This book is dedicated to my husband, Tunis. You are my rock, my love, and my support. And to my children, Karis and Cooper, who inspire me to be a better parent and a better person.

# *Acknowledgments*

I would like to thank those who have guided my education through the years and those who have created in me a desire to help others and a passion for sharing a message of health.

First of all, I thank my parents who taught me to never give up and helped me learn that the squeaky wheel gets the grease (and I am a very squeaky wheel).

I also want to thank my first chiropractor, Dr. Elliot Grusky, who gave me my first adjustment and led me to the path I am on now.

Next I want to thank the ICPA (International Chiropractic Pediatric Association) for all the wonderful doctors and teachers they have brought into my life. They have given to me such a wealth of information that I am excited to share in this book.

Finally I want to thank my husband who knows me so well, understands my passion, and listens to me when I talk (even if for hours on end).

You are just a few of the people in my life who have made me the woman I am today — in the pages of this book I hope you can see how you have inspired me.

# *Contents*

# *Introduction*

This book is about chiropractic care (which will be referred to as simply *chiropractic* from here on) and how you can use it to benefit your life, your children's lives, and your family's lives. I wrote this book because I want to share how beneficial this kind of healthcare can be for everyone. I have the desire to speak to everyone I meet about the benefits of chiropractic healthcare for all ages, from birth to death; but there's not enough time in the day. I hope that this book can do it for me.

My passion for chiropractic began in my teen years. When I was a little girl, I had a lot of pain in my legs, and I suffered through migraine headaches. The pain was severe, and by high school it became intolerable. I saw many doctors.

One doctor said, "She'll be in a wheelchair by the time she's eighteen."

Nobody had any answers. They just kept taking X-rays and prescribing drugs.

Finally, I went to a doctor who shook my hand, looked at my mom, and said, "I think she's a hypochondriac."

I was probably about fourteen years old at the time, and I was in debilitating pain. It was so discouraging.

Around the same time, my brother was playing baseball and he hurt his back.

His baseball coach and trainer said, "You're going to my chiropractor now. Go."

My brother was treated successfully, and my mom said, "This is the one doctor we haven't tried with you. Why don't we go ahead and get you checked out?"

It turns out I had scoliosis.

My chiropractor, Dr. Elliot Grusky, said, "It looks like your neck is on backwards! What's happened to you?"

Since the age of four, I had spent almost every year in a cast of some sort, with various broken bones. I had broken my femur when I was four years old, and spent eight weeks in traction and another eight weeks in a full body cast.

It turns out that spending every spring in a cast of some kind during your formative years does some damage to your spine as you're growing and hobbling along. By fourteen years old, the accumulative damage had created my extreme symptoms.

Within three months of treatment, I was a new person. I felt so much better. I had wanted to become a veterinarian, until that point.

Then I thought: *No, this is what I want to do.*

Nothing was helping until I saw the chiropractor. The medication I had been taking was giving me potential ulcers. With just chiropractic adjustments—nothing else—within three months I went from not being able to do homework without having migraines and passing out, to running up and down the athletic fields.

I told my brother's trainer that I was so grateful for him sending my brother to this chiropractor that I wanted to work with him. Eventually I became an athletic trainer. I won a scholarship to a four-year college for athletic training and graduated early. I then attended massage therapy school, earning a massage therapy license, with the purpose in mind of going to chiropractic school so I could be the best chiropractor I could be.

I wanted to be able to take care of other young people. Chiropractors are trained to recognize that every little bump and bruise along the way can make major effective changes in a growing spine. As parents, if we don't recognize this, we could unintentionally be doing our children a disservice as they get older.

That is a big part of the reason I wrote this book. I wanted to write it so that mothers and fathers can think about how they can benefit their kids in the long run.

It is best to read this book from the beginning. Then you can get a good understanding of what chiropractic is all about, how it relates to the nervous system, and why it's important for treating problems and for preventative care. It is best not to skip the introductory sections so you can get a full understanding before looking up symptoms.

As I tell my children, understanding something is more important than memorizing it. If you understand why you're doing something and how it works, then you own it.

This book is not really about answers, although you will find many as you read; it's more about understanding how important questions are, and about learning how to find the answers you are looking for. It's about getting informed and making informed decisions about your family's healthcare.

*Chapter* **ONE**

# The Nervous System

## HOW THE NERVOUS SYSTEM WORKS

Your nervous system controls all of the functions of your body:

- Your heart can't beat if your nervous system is not working.
- Your legs won't move.
- Food won't digest.

It is the control room of the body; every other function relies on the nervous system.

It is important to understand how the nervous system works. If you don't understand it, how can you know how to help it work properly?

You will learn about the structure and function of the nervous system in this chapter.

**The Nervous System Takes In Information**

From birth to death, your nervous system is what enables you to understand what's happening in your environment.

Using your senses, it takes in:

- Sights
- Sounds
- Smells
- Tastes
- Tactile information

All these sensations are used to help your body make decisions — directing your actions and reactions.

The nervous system takes in information about dangers in your world so that your brain can decide what to do to avoid or combat dangerous situations. It allows you to feel pain so that you can be aware of injury.

When faced with a danger, do you need to walk or run, sit or stand, jump up, or duck down?

Information coming in via the nervous system helps you make these decisions.

You might not realize that your nervous system is also responsible for taking in immunity information so that you can fight off illness and repair injuries. In addition, your nervous system also receives and processes intangible stimuli like love and other emotions.

It doesn't matter if you're a baby or a fully-grown adult; it's this same nervous system that takes in information and processes it in the brain. As you grow, however, you develop learned responses.

If a baby is hungry, they can sense this using their nervous system, but they can't satisfy this need themselves. Their reaction is just to cry and cry until somebody else brings them what they need. An older child will learn to recognize hunger and respond by getting some food.

As you grow, you learn how to adapt; you learn from your mistakes or experiences, and this learning is also directed by the nervous system. You still have the same urges, but as you grow, your ability to respond improves. Basic human nature is the same in everybody. Information from your surroundings is taken in and processed, but it's your experiences, your life experiences, that make your responses different.

## The Nervous System Interprets Information and Responds

The nervous system also has to interpret information after it enters. For example, if you touch a hot pot and the sensory information enters — the skin senses heat and pain in this case — it has to interpret this information correctly:

*Heat and pain means the pot is hot.*

After this, the nervous system needs to direct a response that makes sense:

*That's painful! Move the arm! Move your hand away quickly!*

Both the interpretation and the response need to be correct. Your brain must interpret the sensation of burning and then initiate the correct response. In this case, the response may be so fast that your hand may move before you even think about it. But the nervous system can collect more complicated forms of information that require more thoughtful processing.

For example, if you see a dog when you're out walking, will you pet the dog, or move away?

Your nervous system will take in visual and auditory sensations and will combine this information with memories of past experiences:

*Is the dog showing its teeth?*

*Is the dog growling?*

*Is the dog recognizable as a friendly neighbor, or is it unfamiliar?*

Based on the information collected by the nervous system, your brain can make an appropriate response. Interpreting the data correctly is important and so is quickness of response. This is true of the muscle responses in these examples, but it's also true of immune system responses.

Your immune system needs to function at its highest capacity so that your internal environment can quickly and correctly respond to dangers — breathing in toxins, ingesting a poison, or exposure to a pathogen.

In these cases the nervous system, in cooperation with the immune system, has to interpret the input and produce the right reaction, whether it's sneezing, coughing, fever, or antibody production; whatever response is best to combat the danger.

Your nervous system needs to function as close to maximum efficiency as possible. If it is not functioning properly, your reaction times to dangers will be slow. Slow reactions, as you can imagine, could potentially be life-threatening.

## Voluntary and Involuntary Actions

Your nervous system controls *voluntary actions*. You are consciously aware of these actions and actively *choose* to perform them.

For example, you can choose:

- To run
- To stand up
- To walk
- To sit
- To throw a ball

Your brain makes these choices purposefully and directs the complex muscle actions that will create the movements you want.

Your nervous system also controls *involuntary actions* that you do not have to think about at all.

These kinds of actions are happening every minute of every day, for example:

- Your heart beats
- Your lungs expand and contract
- Your eyes blink
- Your kidneys filter your blood

You don't have to think about these actions. Your body is doing many tasks that you are not aware of, and your nervous system can monitor and react to changes automatically, without any thought. It is clear that the proper functioning of the nervous system is vital to our survival.

The nervous system is like a network; it is like a major city power plant which has its headquarters in the brain. Nerve cells from the brain extend all around the body the same way that wires extend from a power plant through the city to direct various functions.

I like to picture the wires held up on utility poles, or transformers all around the body, with bundles of wires extending from the brain held together in the spinal cord.

From these imaginary utility poles, I picture more wires extending into homes and then continuing into each individual electrical outlet in each room. I think of these rooms as the different body systems, and I think of the outlets as connecting to all the various parts of the body — the heart, the skin, the muscles, and every other organ of the body.

Looking at the structure this way, you can see that the nervous system wiring network is the means by which the central part of the system — the brain and spinal cord — communicates with all of the external systems.

What happens if something goes wrong with this control system?

In this analogy, if the power plant blows up, of course, everything's over; there's no recovering from the destruction of the brain.

What about more minor problems with the system?

Well, if one of those transformers or utility poles is damaged, it may affect one outlet or could set off an entire house or block of houses. Those transformers and poles need to be upright, standing the way they're designed to be. We consider the functioning of the control system when we're faced with problems in our homes.

Going back to our power plant analogy, suppose you try to turn on your television and it doesn't work.

You can keep trying to fix the television, but what if the problem was caused by a car that hit a pole down the road?

You can call an appliance repairman to come fix your television, or you can call an electrician to check your wiring, but you will be wasting your hard-earned money.

Instead, first you'll check that the television is plugged into the outlet, and you'll probably also check other appliances on the same circuit to see if they are working. Eventually, you will see that the power isn't entering your house because of the broken pole.

As chiropractors, we are constantly assessing how the nervous system wiring relates to other complaints.

When a patient comes in with shoulder pain, for instance, a good chiropractor will be alert to the possibility that the nerve supply to the upper back or neck is playing a role in the shoulder issue.

## ADULTS AND CHILDREN: SIMILARITIES AND DIFFERENCES

We are all human beings, but although we share much in common, we are all individuals. No two fingerprints are the same. In addition, we are given choices throughout our lives and the choices we make affect our development. As we mature, our human bodies are all similar, but our choices and our life environment can affect how we grow and change.

### Babies and Children Are Little Versions of Us

This title could be seen as a controversial statement, so first I will explain. When I say that children are little versions of ourselves, I don't mean that we should treat them like adults, but that our basic structure is the same.

We have two eyes, we have four limbs, we have a heart and lungs, and we contain the same organs. Our nervous system function is the same. When injured, the human body of an adult uses the same processes to heal as a baby's body does. You sneeze just like a baby does when you have a cold. Our body's responses to outward influences are the same in the adult and in the child.

## Growth and Development

The ultimate goal of the developmental activities in a little newborn child is to create an adult human. This process depends on the phenomenon of *innate intelligence*—your body's ability to grow, heal, and function without voluntary initiative.

Involuntary responses occur in babies and adults, but the nervous system has a dual function in children—because it also helps direct growth and development. Bones grow longer. Hearts and lungs grow larger.

Each stage of growth requires precise management and proper timing; the process of development from child to adult takes a great deal of organization. When your body reaches adulthood, these functions cease. Your growth phase ends, and your body functions focus on maintenance and survival.

## Interference

I like this saying:

*Nature doesn't need any help. It just needs no interference.*

During development, your body naturally grows and changes. Your heart gets bigger as you grow, your bones get longer, and so on; all of these things will happen as long as there's no interference. As long as the power lines aren't down, as long as the spinal cord, the brain, and all the systems can accomplish what they need to do, these functions will naturally occur.

But what happens when there is interference in the natural processes of the body?

For example, what if the proper timing of bone growth is interfered with?

It is possible that a necessary process in bone development might be cut short. This could result in a misalignment of the spine that causes pressure on the neuromuscular system.

Another kind of interference could cause the immune system to function improperly. If the immune system isn't able to respond quickly, or even at all, this could make the body more susceptible to illness. Interference can cause organs to function inefficiently or improperly.

Interference in the natural processes of development can affect children, leading to symptoms like asthma and inefficient body functioning. Interference in an adult's physiological processes can result in pain and poor health.

One of the goals of chiropractic is to clear away any interference so you can thrive.

## PROPER FUNCTIONING OF THE NERVOUS SYSTEM IN A CHILD'S DAILY LIFE

### The Central and Peripheral Nervous Systems

The *central nervous system* consists of the control centers—the brain and spinal cord. The *peripheral nervous system* carries messages to and from the central nervous system; it sends information to the brain and carries out orders from the brain.

Messages travel through the *cranial nerves*, which branch out from the brain and go to the ears, eyes, and face. Messages also travel through the *spinal nerves*, which branch out from the spinal cord and travel to the rest of the body.

There are two major parts to the peripheral nervous system: the *somatic* system, which is responsible for sensory input and muscle movement, and the *autonomic* system, which is responsible for all the automatic functions, like breathing and digestion.

## Growth and Development

The nervous system helps direct the growth and development of children, not only physically, but also mentally. Each stage of growth is different and involves specific body adaptations.

Newborns cannot hold up their heads, but quickly gain this ability. They progressively learn to roll over, sit, crawl, and walk.

Each stage is an important step in growth, and the order of those stages is important. As you grow bigger and stronger, you move from walking to running, jumping, and so on. You develop hand-eye coordination, balance, complex movements, and the ability to play with others; all of these advances are important.

## Immune Function

Your immune system within your body is always at the ready — ready to fight off invaders. Signals come down through the nervous system to a warehouse of sorts — containing an army of immune fighters.

When an invader enters your body, there are some reflex reactions that can occur, like a sneeze or a cough, but sometimes more specific combat is required.

The immune system might send in a tow truck, but sometimes it might have to send in the Navy SEALs.

The brain and immune system cooperate to make this decision and start the process.

What if there is interference with this process?

If there is interference or improper communication, a delay or an ineffective battle plan may result, or perhaps a lack of response altogether.

When a chiropractor removes that interference, your immune function can once again fight off invaders; it quickly figures out the correct strategy to take.

Sometimes symptoms that we experience are a result of natural, automatic immune functions.

Here are some examples:

- Coughing
- Sneezing
- Fever
- Vomiting
- Diarrhea

These symptoms are proper immune functions. Your body is responding to an attack and fighting off whatever has invaded.

Unfortunately, you don't feel good when these things happen, but they are signals that your body is working, and it's working for you in a positive way. It is important to prevent interference with this system, so that as a baby, child, or adult, you can fight off invaders. You can't prevent all invaders from affecting you. You just need to know how to fight them.

From the brain to the very end of each nerve, it is vital to keep communication lines open and remove any interference for proper function. This is an important focus of chiropractic.

**Body Awareness**

What if you were born in a room with a red light on and a constant buzzing sound?

Imagine this is all you have ever known.

What if someone walked into that room and turned off the red light and turned off that buzzing sound?

Imagine how much clearer your world would be and how much more you could see and hear. In the red buzzing room, you didn't know that your world could be different at all, how much more wonderful things could be.

Would you choose to go back to the buzzing red light room, when you know how clear the world can look?

*Body awareness* refers to how alert you are to the condition of your body. Although your nervous system receives all your sensory information, it is possible that you are not interpreting the information correctly. Chiropractic treatment is designed to help patients accurately assess the health status of their body.

How alert are you to the condition of your body?

Are you healthy?

Do you know what it *feels* like to be healthy?

Imagine that you live next to a train track. Eventually, you get used to that train going by. You don't even notice the train noise.

Then imagine that someone shows up at your house and asks you how you can stand living close to that train and all the noise.

So, you notice the noise again. Having it pointed out to you may make it hard for you to continue ignoring the noise.

In my office, I often witness children who have been feeling discomfort for so long, they didn't know what it felt like to feel good. They had no idea.

They just thought: *This is how life is. I was born with it; this is how it is. This is what it is supposed to feel like.*

These children are sometimes grumpy or moody when I first see them — which is understandable. After their first chiropractic adjustment, sometimes there is a dramatic change; it is like turning off the red light and the buzzing sound. It is like hearing clearly for the first time, or being able to take their first full deep breath.

Besides the sensation of feeling better, there is an additional jolt of surprise that comes from the realization that they were *not* feeling good before, but never knew it.

Being body aware is such a wonderful gift for kids, not only for the present time, but for the future as they grow. They can say to themselves:

*I know what it feels like to feel good.*

More importantly, at times when their health is not flourishing, they will have the ability to say to themselves:

*I know what it feels like to feel good, and this is not right.*

Then they can make good decisions regarding their own health.

They can also realize when their bodies don't feel right and make decisions to fix the problem.

They become educated about their own health by correctly sensing their body reactions:

*When I eat that, it doesn't make me feel good.*

*When I do that, my body hurts afterwards.*

They become able to make decisions, and this ability stays with them as they grow.

Some adults have mistaken expectations regarding aging, and their body awareness suffers as a result. Sometimes patients come in to see me and are certain that their symptoms are due to aging.

Patients may believe that being bloated or experiencing chronic pain are symptoms of aging, and that they will just have to learn with the pain or discomfort.

This belief can be a mistake in their body awareness; sometimes symptoms have nothing to do with aging, but with another problem, like a gluten sensitivity or a postural issue.

After an adjustment and some discussion, often people finally realize that they don't have to feel bad or live with pain. There is regained body awareness. Patients feel what it is like to stand and sit straight and it feels good. It feels *right.*

I often hear comments like, "After you adjusted me, I felt like I sat up straighter, longer. I just felt like I could, but I felt like I had to now, because every time I slouched, it didn't feel right."

This is what it's like to become body-aware. You know what it feels like to be out of sorts, and you know what it is like to feel good. Body awareness is a gift for children, but it's a gift for adults as well.

*Chapter* **TWO**

# Why See a Chiropractor When There is No Pain?

## KIDS ARE RESILIENT—BUT NOT IMMUNE TO INJURY

A lot of people ask why should they bring a child to see a chiropractor if the child isn't in any pain.

Well, you still bring your car in for repairs and maintenance before it falls apart, right?

You still want to get an oil change and a tune up before that "Check Engine" light comes on, don't you?

In the same way, you want to give your body, and your children's bodies, regular checkups and maintenance to keep them working well.

The relationship between pain and chiropractic is misunderstood by many. It is important to recognize that:

- Pain isn't the only factor that determines whether an injury has taken place.

- Chiropractic isn't just about relieving pain.

- Chiropractic is more about preventing pain.

- Chiropractic addresses other symptoms besides pain.

- Pain can be misleading.

- Hidden issues may remain when pain disappears.

- Unaddressed injuries can have a cumulative effect.

- Sometimes children's injuries go unnoticed because they are so resilient.

If an adult fell down the stairs in your home, you would be quick to assess for injury, but if a child fell down the stairs, you may think: *Oh, brush it off, you'll be okay.*

Children trip. They fall. They bump their heads. You want them to get up and move on, but sometimes you try to convince yourself that they are more resilient than they are.

The reality is, yes, they bounce back quickly. They have a shorter distance to fall than you do as an adult, but it is a mistake to keep telling them to ignore pain that they have when they have an accident. Teaching kids to ignore how they feel, to ignore their pain, is not wise.

Yes, they can get up and move around, and they're not as debilitated as adults after a fall. But maybe they are showing signs of pain in different ways.

If your child falls, she doesn't have to cry about it all day, but you need to recognize that an injury happened. Injuries can lead to other problems, even if the child is not expressing pain, even if she's not limping, even if she's still able to use the arm that she fell on. Just because a kid isn't complaining about pain for a week doesn't mean that there is no problem to address.

Addressing the little injuries that children have can potentially help them later when they become adults. Sometimes a series of unaddressed little injuries can combine to make a difficult problem to fix in an adult.

## A Child's Growing Body Heals Fast

Because they're growing, children's bones heal faster. They are going to recover faster than adults, because there are more growing and healing receptors in their body.

So, when a kid tumbles down the stairs, you can hug them and hold them, let them cry a little, dust them off, and send them on their way, knowing they're going to start healing quickly. But you know if you fell down the stairs, you'd be out of commission for quite a while.

So while you need to assess if there is any serious injury that needs to be addressed when a child falls, it is true that their bodies do have the ability to heal remarkably fast.

## THE UNKNOWN SYMPTOMS

### Pain Can Show Up as Anger and Frustration

Pain is just a symptom, but it is an important one to understand. When you are talking about children's pain, you need to understand the symptom from a child's point of view.

How does pain manifest in a child?

What do they feel?

How do they communicate?

A child will not express themselves like an adult. They may be too young to communicate in words at all. They may not comprehend the sensations they are experiencing. Inside, perhaps their little mind might only understand pain to this extent:

*What is this feeling I have?*

*I don't know, but I need it to stop!*

A young child who can't express these feelings may show these reactions:

- Crying
- Anger
- Head-banging
- Hitting themselves
- Hitting others
- Acting out in frustration

As an adult, pain may make you grumpy or moody or snippy, but you know how to express your feelings and socially interact with other people. You can understand what you are feeling and can reason out a way to deal with your pain, but babies can't be reasoned with. They don't understand, so it is up to adults to figure out what they are feeling.

Let's not forget the possibility of spinal misalignments that can cause interference later on. When a child has a big fall it is best to have a chiropractor evaluate him or her.

I've had child patients who have come into my office grumpy and silent. Sometimes they've been hitting others at school, and a parent had been asked to pick them up from school because of this.

If I suggest an adjustment, parents often don't have any confidence that this will help, but wish me luck as I give it a try.

It is gratifying to experience a successful adjustment and have a child look up in surprise and say, "Ah, that feels better."

Children often don't know what's going on inside their own bodies. They can't ask for an adjustment or even vocalize that they do not feel well or right.

When we adjust children, regardless of whether or not they have pain, we're able to remove interference. It is especially rewarding to be able to remove symptoms that they're not able to express that they have.

## Developmental Issues and Misalignment

Why should you bring your child to a chiropractor?

It might surprise you to know that there are developmental issues that can be expressed as a misalignment in the spine.

Consider these questions:

- Does your child have trouble seeing the board at school?
- Does your child have trouble hearing?
- Is your child having difficulty learning to read?

- Is your child having learning difficulties?
- Is your child acting out because of frustration?
- Is your child having difficulty with speech?
- Are motor skills delayed or awkward?
- Is your child experiencing undue aches and pains during normal activity?

Besides the last item on the list — pain — parents are often not aware of the many difficulties that a chiropractor can address for children.

It has been shown that problems with vision, which a child might convey by saying he can't see the board at school, can be the result of a misalignment.

Does this surprise you?

The first recorded successful chiropractic adjustment was in 1895 on a man named Harvey Lillard. Mr. Lillard had been deaf for seventeen years and after an adjustment — which may have corrected a spinal nerve misplacement — he was able to hear again.

I'm not promising that every adjustment is going to make deaf people hear and blind people see. However, there are a lot of misalignments in the spine that can lead to interference in areas of body functioning that seem unrelated; in vision, in hearing, in ability to read or comprehend, in speech, and in other areas.

Sometimes the interference has been caused by adverse trauma, or misalignments to the spine. We are able to address those issues simply and noninvasively, especially when they are caught early.

If your child is having issues like this, why don't you check with a chiropractor and see if they're able to help you?

## Babies and Head Shaping

Babies sometimes suffer problems such as misshapen heads or flattened skulls that a chiropractor can help address. Leaving these structural issues untreated can lead to other issues down the line, including developmental interference issues. This topic will be further addressed in the section on *torticollis* in Chapter Four.

## Gait Issues—Delayed or Improper Crawling and Walking

You might think that the way your children get around—their gait—in the early days doesn't matter, but it does matter. It matters a great deal.

Below are three important gait issues in child development. Each will be discussed further:

- Your child should be crawling first, before they walk.
- Crawling should be on hands and knees.
- Walking should involve a *heel-toe* motion of the foot.

Many parents think that getting from Point A to Point B is the only developmental issue they should be concerned about, but this is not so.

Crawling properly means the child is on hands and knees, moving forward, using all four limbs. This is not the same as scooting on their bottom or moving forward using one side and dragging the other. It's not the same as an army crawl or belly crawl.

Why is proper crawling so important?

The development of proper crawling technique is important for these reasons:

- These motions impact the functional development of the spine.

- Proper crawling helps create the *lordosis* — the scooping curve in your low back — that a baby needs for proper development of the lumbar area.

- Crawling also helps create the curvature of the cervical spine in the neck, making sure that heads look up while the tail is dropping down.

- Proper crawling helps the process of developing hand-eye coordination.

- The *cross-crawl pattern* — right arm and left leg, followed by the reverse — allows the brain to practice coordinating the workings of the right and left sides of the brain. This right-left brain coordination will become important for many brain processes.

- Crawling strengthens the spine.

- Crawling *before* walking enables the spine to become strong enough to be able to sustain a standing, walking position.

Walking gait is also very important in a child's development.

Young children learning to walk will be flat-footed for a while. But as they gain balance and stability and learn to run, they will move with a heel-toe, heel-toe pattern. They should not be walking on their toes or flat-footed. Their knees should be bending during the walking motion. Not developing a good stride can result in interference with other body processes resulting in problems, including digestive issues and learning difficulties.

So, what should you do if your child doesn't crawl, but goes straight to walking?

And what can you do if your child isn't crawling or walking properly?

See a chiropractor. A chiropractor can help assess your child's movements and can also educate you on proper exercises to help your child's development.

## CHIROPRACTORS ARE PREVENTATIVE DOCTORS

The goal of a chiropractor is to facilitate the body's ability to heal itself.

By facilitating the body's own abilities, we aim:

- To help the body fight off disease
- To repair misalignments and other improperly functioning elements
- To prevent further damage
- To remove interfering influences
- To assist the body in functioning efficiently

Unfortunately, there are some healthcare professionals who are *only* looking at disease, and so, they really can only help when you are sick. Detection can be valuable; medical doctors have wonderful tools for detection, but chiropractors are really in the business of prevention. Just like you brush your teeth to prevent cavities, under chiropractic care, you get adjustments to prevent your body's inability to function.

## Adjustments Boost the Immune System

Many fighters live in your body. They can be found in your gut, in your blood, and in many different organs. Think of them like the army, the marines, the coast guard, the navy — all staying at the ready to fight any invaders that come in. The brain directs the fighters, deciding which department of defense needs to be sent.

When you have interference in your nervous system and an invading attacker comes in — whether it's a virus, fungus, or bacteria — the connection is interrupted. The defenders are unable to fight to the best of their ability.

If there's static on the line, the message won't get through; perhaps the fighters won't know what to do. They won't know how to respond.

They'll wonder how to deal with the invasion:

*Who do we send?*

*How many of them?*

*How fast?*

Perhaps they can't get that information out fast enough, and their response is delayed. Perhaps they get the message wrong.

Chiropractic can help to clear the interference. When a chiropractor does this, it doesn't mean that you're never going to get sick. It just means that when an invader comes in, the system doesn't have to navigate around an interference — your body will be at the ready to defend and ward off illness as quickly and efficiently as possible.

I have noticed in my practice that children who get regular adjustments don't miss school much for being sick. I define *sickness* specifically; true *sickness* only occurs when your body is not performing proper body functions to expel an invader, or is feeling unwell.

Symptoms of sickness include:

- Lethargy
- High fever
- Lack of urine
- Dehydration
- Lack of sweating with a fever

In contrast, you may sometimes feel a little off, but this is not necessarily a sickness. It is important to distinguish between your normal body functioning and genuine sickness.

Remember, what we think of as symptoms are reactions, or evidence that your body is functioning the way it should:

- Fever
- Cough
- Sneeze
- Diarrhea
- Vomiting

These reactions don't mean that you are sick; they mean that your body is doing what it needs to do—sending out warriors to push the invaders back out.

I don't use the word *sick* in this case; instead, I think: *You don't feel well.*

When your child doesn't feel well, you might keep them home; but they should bounce right back.

I've noticed that children—including my own—who get adjusted more regularly don't get sick as much as those who are not getting adjusted regularly. Your chiropractor can also talk with you about proper nutrition, which benefits the adjustment, to make sure that your body knows how to regulate itself.

## We Correct Misalignments to Prevent Further Pain or Issues

After you drive a brand new car off the lot, you still bring it in every three thousand miles to get an oil change. You still get the tires aligned.

You brush your teeth and take your kids to the dentist every few months to get teeth checked and cleaned to prevent cavities.

In the same way, ideally, children should be adjusted regularly for their best health through all developmental stages and whenever a significant health event has occurred.

For example:

- In the earliest stages, I examine babies and encourage them to learn to hold their head up.

- When they start crawling, I see them again to assess their movement.

- Children should come in again to be assessed when they start walking.

- When teeth start coming in, they should be examined.

- If a child gets braces, or has other work done on the teeth, they should come in.

- And, of course, a child should be seen whenever an injury has occurred.

At each stage they should be coming to get adjusted, to make sure that their body remains balanced.

As discussed before, when we treat kids, they become body-aware. They understand how their bodies are supposed to feel so they can learn to be aware when problems arise. Hopefully, we parents can do the one thing that we all want: teach our kids not to make our mistakes.

Children have to learn some things on their own; you can't teach them everything, but you can start them off the right way. If we can treat kids now, maybe we can raise a generation of kids who don't have old-man and old-lady pains.

Maybe the next generation won't be repeating:

"Oh, that's my back, it's just hurting because I'm getting old."

"My knees hurt; I guess I'm just getting old."

Most important, you need to teach children what it feels like to feel awesome, so that they can grow up to make decisions to continue to feel awesome.

Let's start them off knowing what a healthy body feels like:

*This is how I feel good, and this is what makes me feel bad.*

From there they will know how to make proper choices. If they don't know what feels good and what feels bad, they will have no good way to make decisions. But with the knowledge that body awareness gives them, they can assess all of their other choices:

*When I eat this, I feel good.*

*When I eat that, I feel bad.*

*When I get adjusted, I feel good.*

*When I don't get adjusted, I feel bad.*

And so on. If they don't have that frame of reference, how can they learn to make good choices as they get older?

## Chiropractors Facilitate the Body's Ability to Heal and Grow

Nature does not need any help. It simply requires no interference. If there is no interference, your body has the ability to perform every function perfectly. If you remove interference by getting adjustments regularly, then you will be able to grow and be the most awesome self you can be.

I have a young patient who first came in after having five recent ear infections and had other health issues as well. After getting regular adjustments and using natural remedies, he now feels awesome.

He had not been listening to his body; he just wasn't paying attention. After we started clearing away issues, we realized he couldn't hear—he had heavy, chronic wax buildup.

In addition, he had taken many antibiotics, and they had upset the natural balance of his digestive system. He had little appetite and ate large amounts of sugary foods and dairy, which further debilitated his digestive tract by feeding the bacteria that was overgrowing in his body.

Once we cleared the imbalance of good bacteria in his body, he felt awesome. When he comes in for his adjustments now, it's wonderful to see how happy he is. His sister is a patient of mine as well. The family is happier as a whole, and they have come to understand that they all feel better when they come for regular adjustments.

Have you ever heard the saying, "early detection is key"?

Who needs detection when you can have prevention?

Certainly, the early detection slogan applies to mammograms and breast cancer and there's nothing wrong with monitoring your body, but my goal is to raise generations of kids who don't have to suffer from the pains that we have. My goal is prevention.

I want to help people understand how to make good choices, from healthcare to nutrition. We cannot continue in the cycle of ignorance. We can help prevent so many health problems if we educate ourselves and our children.

*Chapter* **THREE**

# How to Choose a Chiropractor

## GETTING REFERRALS

Have you decided to see a chiropractor?

Getting a referral is a great idea: you're confident in your choice and don't waste a lot of your time. When you have a referral from someone you trust, you avoid an appointment with a complete stranger. Before you start, you have the opportunity to get to know that person through someone else.

### Talk to Friends and Family

When you are researching chiropractors, you can certainly go on the Internet and find someone who has an office as close to you as possible, but I feel it is best to get recommendations from people you trust.

Here are some people to start with:

- Friends
- Co-workers
- Family members
- Neighbors

Ask them whom they go to for chiropractic care, whether they like that practitioner, and what they experienced during visits and alignments.

If you have found a chiropractor who interests you on the Internet, ask around about them before you make an appointment.

Use social media and social networking sites like Facebook or Twitter to research. On Facebook, I am a member of some groups that are designed for local people, like mom networking and natural parenting. Look for groups in your local area and post questions on those pages; you might receive helpful answers.

Some responses will be specific referrals with names and locations of a chiropractor. You might also find others who are searching for care and willing to join you on the journey.

In my practice, I probably have at least three to four patients a week coming straight from referrals on social media. One day, seven new patients visited who had found my practice by asking online for recommendations. You will also find sites that have health professionals as members and welcome questions about health and disease. I'm a part of some of those groups as well.

Social media provides an opportunity to ask other questions of people who go to chiropractors. You can ask questions about how appointments are structured and about other people's experience with procedures. Getting a little bit of information before your appointment can give you more peace of mind before you walk in to meet a stranger.

## The International Chiropractic Pediatric Association

The International Chiropractic Pediatric Association (ICPA) is an international organization for chiropractors who work with children. You can find more information about ICPA at www.icpa4kids.com.

Perhaps someone has recommended that you take your child to a chiropractor, but you feel you need more information before you commit to this idea?

The ICPA website is an excellent resource for you.

Suppose you are looking for a chiropractor in Orlando, Florida?

The ICPA is an international organization with listings of doctors; check the website and for someone who matches your needs and expectations.

Suppose you have questions about particular topics.

Search the ICPA website for information in many areas and explore different kinds of research.

The ICPA is an association meant to advance the chiropractic family and wellness lifestyle. It's an organization that provides a place where you can find chiropractors, but is also an organization where chiropractors go to learn.

Doctors who are part of an ICPA program have taken time to not only join the program, but also have taken time to learn from experienced doctors in a standardized manner. If you move from one state to another and need to change chiropractors, you can go onto the ICPA website and know you will be able to find someone near your new home who uses similar methods and are trained in various areas such as the Webster Technique, used specifically during pregnancy.

The ICPA is also a great place to find research that any layperson, like a parent, can access. You access the site and search for information and research on particular topics.

For example, if your child has chronic ear infections, you can search that topic and learn what kind of research has been done regarding pediatric chiropractic care. The ICPA is a resource to not only help you find a chiropractor, but a resource to help answer some questions that you have.

## Talk to Your Current Chiropractor About Treating Your Children

It is easy to find adults who see chiropractors regularly.

However, when I ask them about bringing their children, they often are surprised at the question: "If you are a chiropractic patient, why aren't your children?"

From what you've already read in this book you know I strongly encourage families to bring their children in for adjustments, but it is true that not every chiropractor works with kids. Some, like me, not only work with children, but have a strong focus on them.

Be assured that every chiropractor has learned, at some point, how to adjust a child, but that may not be their focus. Chiropractors specialize in many different areas.

If you want to find a chiropractor who will work with your child, start by asking your current chiropractor these questions:

- Do you adjust kids?
- Would you be willing to look at my child?
- These are the issues I have with my kid. Suggestions?

They might immediately offer to schedule an appointment, or they may refer you to a local colleague.

It isn't necessary to find a different chiropractor just for your kids if your current chiropractor is willing. I adjust adults and children, and I am happy to work with whole families. A lot of people don't realize that; they think you have to find someone who only adjusts kids.

Don't be afraid to ask other people for referrals as well. There are a lot of patients who have had wonderful experiences and who really do want to share about their great chiropractor. You'll meet people who are excited to talk about their awesome experience at their chiropractor's office. Talk to them and hear their stories.

## FINDING A CHIROPRACTOR WHO FITS YOUR FAMILY

If you don't like Indian food, you don't go to an Indian restaurant. If you don't like Mexican food, don't go to a Mexican restaurant.

This makes sense, right?

But many people don't have the same kind of sense about their health professionals. Spend some time and effort to choose the health professionals you really want.

Make sure that when you walk in to any healthcare provider's office — it doesn't matter what kind of provider — to remember that you are hiring them to do a job *for* you. If you are not comfortable with that person from start to finish, then it is okay to find somebody else. That's the bottom line. Make sure you're comfortable with them.

## Interview Your Doctors — Make Sure They're a Good Fit

We have a lot of patients in my pediatric and prenatal practice who make new patient appointments and are ready to get started. A lot of those patients have already done their pre-work. They've researched through social media, they've talked to their friends, or they're coming in because of a referral.

Most people who come to me have already heard good things about me or my practice and are ready to begin immediately.

Some patients haven't had a referral but found my name, hand their insurance card over, and ask to start.

Great. It can work like that sometimes. I'm willing to get started and move ahead.

But it's also okay to come into my office, shake my hand, and ask to talk. You are welcome to see how I interact with your children before you decide.

If you do this, however, make sure you set it up ahead of time.

Call the chiropractor's office in advance ask for a consultation appointment, to ensure the proper time and setting are set aside for your visit. Most doctors do a free consultation and will give you an opportunity to determine that you fit together well.

When you arrive, let the doctors and the staff know from the beginning that you desire a consultation. Fill out the paperwork but indicate that you will not schedule care until you have determined if this doctor is the proper fit.

Remember, the doctor should value your time as much as you value theirs.

You need to make sure your child is comfortable with the doctor as well. Children have their own biases and preferences. If your child has issues with men, and you make an appointment with a male doctor who is excellent, the relationship won't work because your child isn't comfortable.

If your child has an issue with women with long hair, or someone who wears glasses, you might have to take this into account.

Is this a practice where doctors wear lab coats?

If a small child had a bad experience at a different doctor's' office where all the professionals wore lab coats, you might want to consider this when making your decision.

When you go to visit, examine the office carefully and ask questions.

- What is the atmosphere in the office?
- Is it child-friendly?
- Are you taking your toddler to a sports chiropractic office where there are no toys?
- Try to see the office and the personnel from your child's point of view.
- Does the doctor engage your child with a smile and an easy-going manner?
- Does the doctor take time to explain policies and procedures?
- What techniques does the doctor use?
- What training does the doctor have?

- Do the doctor and the staff seem willing to spend time answering your questions?
- Do you feel comfortable?

If the doctor does not engage your child in a friendly way, or the environment is not child-friendly, then maybe that's not the right practice for your child.

Make sure that the office has comfortable surroundings. If you are not comfortable on your first visit, you might consider coming back another day. Everyone has bad days, and every office can have an uncomfortable moment.

If your child seems uncomfortable, but you think they might only need another visit, it's okay to suggest returning on an additional day to continue the consultation.

If you are sure that the office is not for you, then thank the staff for their time and information and tell them you are continuing your search.

## Find a Chiropractor Who's Not Too Far Away

For effective chiropractic, you may need appointments a couple of times per week. At the very least, you'll be there a couple of times per month. You want to choose a practice that isn't too far away from your home.

You may think that it doesn't matter. If you like a doctor, you may be willing to drive some distance.

But think carefully about this.

Are you willing to drive there when your kids are in school, and you've got to get them to other activities too?

Are you considering traffic and weather issues, as well as your work schedule?

Driving far never works out. You won't want to drive forty-five minutes to go see your doctor three days a week.

My pediatrician and my general practitioner can be up to thirty minutes away, but I only go there rarely. My holistic dentist is almost an hour away, but I go there only twice a year. My chiropractor, however, I see at least once a month, occasionally two or three times a week, depending on the issue.

To keep your stress level as a parent as low as possible, it is best to try to find someone located close to your job, work, school, or home. There are many great chiropractors out there. Try to find someone whose hours and location work with your life schedule.

**Personality Matters**

Be sure that the chiropractor you choose has a personality that is a good fit and is someone who understands your family. Also be sure that you're comfortable with the techniques your doctor employs.

As I mentioned earlier, make sure that the environment is kid-friendly and your children are comfortable with the doctor.

If you are seeking a sports chiropractor for your child, be sure to ask if the doctor sees children and provides a child-friendly environment.

Doctors have different personalities. Some doctors talk a lot; some don't. Some have a dry sense of humor, and some are full of fun. Doctors apply different strategies with children.

When I walk in the room, I don't wear a lab coat, and I immediately get on the floor with the kids. That's how I present myself. The kids do not sit on a paper-laden table. We sit on the floor and talk, because I feel it's important to be at their eye level.

When they see how I'm behaving and know I'm not going to to hurt them, half the time they'll climb into my lap so we can talk that way, before we get started.

I let parents and children know clearly from the beginning what is going to happen each step of the way during an adjustment:

"You're going to hear noises, now."

"We're going to move your leg this way now."

And before we do *anything*, I ask:

"Does anyone have any questions? Mom? Dad? Little one?"

I make it clear that I want to know if anybody is apprehensive about any step. We have lots of toys, and we allow children to bring toys. We even demonstrate adjustments on dolls; that's the kind of environment we have.

I have children myself, so I am comfortable with kids. I strive to provide an environment that is the right fit for parents and children.

Don't forget that your chiropractor, your dentist, and your doctor *work for you*. You have the right to move forward into a relationship, or decide not to. In the same way you wouldn't go to a restaurant if you had bad service, don't go to a health professional if you don't feel comfortable with that person or staff.

You have the right to choose what's right for you.

## WHAT TO EXPECT

I would never want to walk into a healthcare situation without knowing what to expect. After you've talked to your friends, family, and co-workers, and found a chiropractor you are willing to see and think will fit your family, you want to know what to expect when you arrive.

If you have no experience with chiropractic treatment, it is helpful to learn what it's all about, especially if you are intending to bring your child.

### How Does a Chiropractor Examine Babies?

If you brought your baby in to see me for adjustment, you'd first see me holding and cuddling your baby. I always stroke a baby's skin. Skin-on-skin contact is an important facet of the process.

During an examination of an infant, I will:

- Look at the shape of the skull
- Put my hands in the baby's mouth
- Look in the baby's eyes
- Check to see if the baby's eyes are tracking properly
- Look in the baby's ears and check for ear infections
- Check for lip ties and tongue ties

- Do some neurological assessments
- Check for reflexes

You may find that your chiropractor performs many of the same tests that your pediatrician does.

In addition, one of the techniques that a chiropractor may use to test for structure and alignment is to hold your baby upside down. This is a momentary action just for newborns and infants. You will be right there with your baby the whole time; actually, sometimes we hold the baby right over Mommy, over pillows.

Not every doctor uses this technique, but it is common with doctors trained in the ICPA. Babies love it. If they are crying, sometimes they will stop. The position balances out the cerebrospinal fluids, but it also gives us directions to misalignments.

The other procedure a chiropractor will likely perform is look at the baby from the bottom, pulling down or taking off their diaper, and looking at their bottom, using a technique called the *Logan Basic*, which enables the chiropractor to align their spine from the bottom up.

So we work both from the top down, and from the bottom up.

## What Is an Adjustment Like for a Baby?

When adjusting a baby — an infant or newborn baby — we don't use the same techniques or amount of pressure used to adjust an adult.

When we adjust adults, we hear *cavitations* — sounds created by air release. We hear noises that are often described as cracks and pops.

When we adjust babies, infants, and toddlers, we don't hear sounds as often because they have more space between their joints. However, when there is a major misalignment, you might hear a small sound.

It is important to realize that for baby alignments we use only a *tiny amount of pressure*; no more pressure than you would use to push on a tomato without breaking the skin. This technique is completely different than the pressure we use with adults.

As your child gets older, the techniques used for adjusting will change.

## Informed Consent: Benefits, Risk, and Alternatives

I believe in informed consent. Your doctor should tell you the benefits, risks, and alternatives of care every step of the way.

With that in mind, if you have any questions before moving further, don't hesitate to ask your doctor:

- Why are you doing this?
- What is it for?
- What does it mean?
- What result will it produce?

But there is a balance. Once you find a doctor whom you trust, that balance is also important. If you have an underlying trust in your doctor, you will be able to trust their training, experience, and expertise so you can allow them to perform the job that you've hired them to do.

In addition, don't let your insurance dictate where you take your child for healthcare. It is unfortunate that although you may be insured for chiropractic, not every insurance company will pay for chiropractic treatment for children.

Most health insurance is not focused on *health*, but on *sickness*, so many won't pay for wellness care or maintenance. Don't let this *sick*-care insurance dictate your *health*-care. If you are aiming for health and wellness for your children, you cannot rely on sick-care insurance to cover that. Make your own healthcare savings account. Don't make decisions entirely based on whether your insurance will cover the cost of the care.

Check with chiropractors about the cost of their care. I have a special rate for children because I believe in healthcare for children and don't want them to have to use their sick-care insurance. I know other chiropractors have similar policies.

*Chapter* **FOUR**

# Chiropractors and Common Family Health Issues

*Note: The intention of this chapter is not to diagnose any symptoms. It is meant to describe symptoms that could be causing issues, and how a chiropractor can help alleviate these symptoms.*

## EARACHES AND EAR INFECTIONS

Ear pain in children is probably the most common health issue that parents contend with. All parents will at some point have a child experiencing an earache. Ear pain does not always mean an ear infection is present, so an examination is important. Also, be aware that when ear infections do exist, they are often caused by viruses, which are not affected by antibiotics. Antibiotics are only effective against bacterial infections.

Your chiropractor can look into your child's ears and evaluate whether or not it is an ear infection, and then adjust to give your child relief. We can also recommend natural remedies to continue healing of your child, no matter what the situation is.

**Sometimes an Earache Is Not an Ear Infection**

An ear infection may present with these kinds of symptoms in a young child:

- Crying
- Pulling at ears
- Moodiness
- Fever
- Putting hands in the mouth
- Drooling
- Vomiting
- Diarrhea
- Redness in ear canal

However, when a child is teething, they may present with the same symptoms, even redness in the ear canal. When looking in the child's ear, it's not uncommon to see redness and irritation simply from teething. With teething comes excessive saliva that is full of enzymes, which further contributes to tissue irritation. In addition, during the teething stages, the child's jaw is being re-shaped, which can cause discomfort.

Your doctor will examine your child's ear thoroughly and also check for other signs—feeling the gums for tenderness in their mouth, checking for distinctive redness on the gum line—to tell if the symptoms are likely to be caused more from teething than not.

## What Can Your Chiropractor Do to Help Your Child's Ear Problems?

During the early stages of life, ear pain can be caused by the physiological process necessary to cut teeth and change the shape of the child's jaw and head to prepare for the new set of teeth.

This re-shaping of their head and jaw creates physiological changes in the body, which also can create a fever. The re-shaping of the jaw creates a new alignment; the mouth has to change shape. This can cause pressure that triggers babies to pull at their ears and put their hands in their mouths.

By adjusting the child using chiropractic techniques, we can give the child relief from these symptoms.

The structure of a child's *eustachian tubes* may make recurring earaches more likely. These passages run from the middle ears to the back of the throat to allow for drainage and equalization. Pressure put on these tubes can cause ear pain, and can result in a true ear infection as well.

In an adult, the tubes are almost vertical, but a child's tubes are more at a forty-five-degree angle. This angle make drainage less efficient. When drainage is slow, the possibility of fluids backing up increases, which creates an environment that lends to infection. Sometimes sleeping in odd positions—like when a sleeping child's head is tilted in a car seat—can cause additional pressure on the eustachian tubes, which can make the situation worse.

When an infection does develop, treatment can be used to end the infection, but it isn't going to keep more from occurring. As chiropractors, we remove the interference so that proper drainage can occur.

Whether or not your doctor diagnoses an ear infection, it is important to get your child adjusted. You may choose to administer antibiotics that your doctor may or may not prescribe. Adding an adjustment to the course of treatment can ease symptoms as well as help prevent further ear problems.

Bring your children for treatment early; don't wait until their situation is chronic. I once worked with a young patient who had been suffering chronic ear infections. When his parents finally brought him in to see me, he had several ear infections within a few years.

With only one adjustment, he was feeling better.

We continued to treat him a little bit longer to remove the interference and allow his body to heal. If you bring a child in at their first ear infection, it takes less time to resolve issues than if you wait until after their fourth or fifth infection.

## Natural Solutions

Instead of putting children on an antibiotic, quite often a simple adjustment combined with some natural supplements can offer relief pretty quickly.

One natural solution is using an olive oil and raw garlic mixture directly in the ears, as garlic is a natural antibiotic. You will want the garlic to be fresh and chopped. Extract the oils from the fresh garlic into a little bit of olive oil; one small clove per tablespoon of olive oil. Less might be required — feel it out for yourself.

Bring the olive oil to body temperature. I put hot water in a larger container, and then put the garlic oil in a little glass container submerged in the hot water.

The garlic and olive oil mixture should be heated to body temperature, not any warmer. Room temperature will feel too cold. You never want to heat the oil directly, because it changes the properties of the oil, and *you never want to risk getting it to be a temperature that is too hot.*

If you create a body temperature mixture, babies and children won't even know you're putting it in their ear. If it's colder, especially if they have a mild fever, they're going to be irritated by the cold sensation in their ear. You can use your pinky finger to apply the garlic oil mixture into your child's ear. *Avoid using any foreign objects in your child's ear.* Your pinky finger should fit comfortably.

You can also purchase a garlic and olive oil mixture at natural, whole food stores, already pre-made. I prefer to make my own, because I know it's fresh, and I know exactly what's in it. When you buy it over the counter, it can be great, but it will have more preservatives in it.

If you are breastfeeding, you may also use breast milk in the ear as another great natural remedy. If you have an older child at home with an ear infection but you are nursing a two-month old, you can still use that breast milk in your older child's ear.

Some more regular maintenance can prevent chronic earaches:

- Make sure ears are cleaned regularly so that they don't have a buildup of wax.

- Make sure that your child is not spending too much time sleeping in a sitting-up position with their head bobbing over.

- Make sure they have the opportunity to lay flat on their back, stomach, or side to allow their head to create a good range of motion.

- Talk to your chiropractor about natural remedies; something that can be used along with whatever you choose to do with your pediatrician.

When you are deciding what to do for your child's health issues, make informed decisions. Ask questions and do research. You should know all your options regarding treatment for any condition, including earaches and ear infections. In the best case scenario, parents, pediatricians, and chiropractors work together for the best outcome.

Interestingly, I've had a pediatrician (who grades ear infections on a scale of one to five, five being the worst) say to me that if an infection is between a one and a two-and-a-half, he sends them to the chiropractor first to see them for two weeks, have them look in their ears, and do some natural remedies. If it's from a two-and-a-half to five, he prescribes antibiotics—which they take to prevent any hearing loss or any other serious issues—however, he still sends them to the chiropractor while they are under the antibiotic care.

No matter whom you see, remember to insist on being well-informed as to treatments, diagnoses, and alternatives.

## DIGESTION

### Spitting Up

Most parents have to deal with children who spit up on occasion. Some children spit up right after eating and others have issues later. Some spit up after eating too fast. Some respond to jostling — like when Daddy grabs the baby right after he finished eating and throws him up in the air. Well, yes, that's going to happen.

But there are kids who spit up constantly.

They live in a bib, and parents can't hand them over to grandpa who doesn't want spit-up on his shirt.

Many issues can be resolved easily and naturally with an adjustment, with some supplementation, but the reality is that some children are just what we call *spitters*. What we need to do is understand this tendency, and how it affects them further down the road.

What would a chiropractor do for a spitter?

I would do the following for a baby with this problem:

- Make an appointment for an adjustment.
- Evaluate the spine.
- Check the baby for a *hiatal hernia* which could be causing a problem.
- Establish whether the baby is eating too much at one time.

- Establish if the baby eats too fast.
- If the baby is breastfed, determine if the milk being let down too fast.
- Assess whether the baby has a sensitivity or an allergy.
- Recommend that the child and mother be put on probiotics.

Typically, once they're put on probiotics, most children resolve the majority of their spitting issues. Adjustments are definitely important as well to make sure that some kind of interference in the nervous system is not the cause of the spitting up problem.

With these strategies, chiropractors often resolve a good portion of spitting up. However, some children might have some residual spitting issues through their infancy. Some children have an extra strong gag reflex and will continue to be spitters to some extent.

## Constipation

Some children have issues with chronic constipation from a young age. Interestingly, in some cases, this tendency seems to be related to spitting issues; sometimes children who were big spitters when they were infants have constipation issues when they are older.

For children who tend to be constipated, the most important treatment is making sure that they are well-hydrated. It is common for parents to misjudge the amount of fluid that children require. You see them drinking juice and milk and eating fruit and you think they are taking in enough, but in reality, they often are not.

An important thing to realize is that by the time they say they are thirsty, *it's already too late*. They're starting to get dehydrated.

Children who are running around and playing at home, outside with friends, and at preschool may not be getting enough water. And they need water. Juice is not water. Milk is not water. Our bodies are made up mostly of water and that's what you need to give your children to keep them hydrated. Before every meal or snack, they should drink four to eight ounces of water, depending on their age, and more during the day when they are active.

Kids will say they're hungry, and they want a snack. When they ask for that snack, hand them some water to drink first.

At dinner, give them water first.

Children's snacks are often loaded with grains and sugars, which compact in their systems, creating a bacterial overload. Instead of continually filling their bellies with food, we need to give them a probiotic to help break down what's in their gut and to ensure they drink enough water.

Children who are constantly constipated are typically picky eaters. They are often sugar seekers and the bacteria in their systems depend on these sugars. Reduce the simple sugars in their diet, including in their drinks. They need to reduce or eliminate juices, and add water, water, water.

To summarize:

- Keep children well-hydrated. Drink water before every meal and throughout the day.
- Reduce carbohydrate intake if it is excessive.
- Reduce sugar intake, including fruit juices.
- Add probiotics to their diet.
- See a chiropractor for adjustment.

## How Your Chiropractor Can Help

If your child has constipation issues, chiropractic adjustment is a must. Constipation is a symptom of interference to the digestive system, to the peristalsis that creates the movement of the gut. Active children are walking, running, falling, and playing on their bikes. These kinds of activities can potentially create misalignment, creating interference to the gut. Adjustment can bring relief in the first appointment.

I have a policy when children come in my office with constipation issues: The bathroom must be kept open when I adjust those children, or a parent needs to bring in a couple of extra diapers.

Typically, after one adjustment for these children who have constipation issues the constipation resolves itself. Sometimes with babies, we will make sure they are wearing a clean diaper, adjust them, and then within a few minutes they'll need a new one.

Even with older kids, quite often we can have immediate relief in that moment. Now this isn't a cure; it takes a little more time for long-term healing. But a child who hasn't gone in days may all of a sudden have relief after one good adjustment. The adjustment is *so* important to make sure there's no interference, so that everything can work properly.

## TORTICOLLIS

### What Is Torticollis?

*Torticollis* is a strain or spasm in the muscles of the neck. It can occur in babies, children, or adults. Torticollis creates an inability for the person to have a full range of motion in the neck. In an adult, this can be painful and restrictive. In a child, it can be detrimental.

When that inability to have full range of motion in the neck occurs in a young child, it can result in a flattened or misshapen head, because of the pressure they experience by being restricted to laying in one position.

It is something that is often overlooked in children. Parents often don't notice the restricted motion.

You think: *Oh, he just likes to lay like that.*

Or sometimes you might notice what looks like a preference but you don't see it as a potential problem: *She must like that side because she's always turned that way.*

It is something that should be and can be addressed very easily with a chiropractor.

Look for these early symptoms:

- Having consistent difficulty nursing from one side
- Refusal of the bottle when offered from one side
- Showing discomfort lying on one side

**What Causes Torticollis?**

In adults, torticollis can be caused by something transient—perhaps falling asleep with your head crooked over a pillow or overuse of one side of the body. In babies, it actually can be caused at birth from forceps, suction, or even a C-section.

Birth trauma is one of the most common reasons for torticollis in a baby. When occuring at birth, a parent may not recognize this as a problem right away, as I've already stated. Remember that babies should have full range of motion no matter what, and if they don't, see your healthcare professional about this.

Sometimes, whether birth trauma has occurred or not, a baby strongly prefers one side to nurse. Often this is the first sign that there's a problem. If you notice this, it is important to let your doctors know.

Sometimes infants will only nurse when facing in one direction; if you turn them around they resist nursing. If you are bottle feeding, when you hold the bottle up, they perhaps don't turn their head towards it except from one side. Parents might tend to allow them to have that favoritism, which is not recommended. You want to make sure they have full range of motion as they are growing.

Extreme torticollis issues, if left untreated, can lead to misshapen heads, vision and hearing problems, and learning difficulties down the road.

If the child's head is turned too far to the right or left, the result is an inability to see out of both eyes when he is looking straight ahead.

A child with this problem is not getting full use out of both eyes and both ears. They're going to be unbalanced, with one eye stronger than the other, and one ear stronger than the other. In addition, more ear infections are possible with a child with long-term torticollis.

As a parent, make sure you address and resolve torticollis issues quickly.

## How Your Chiropractor Can Help

We can help not only through adjustments — which arc always gentle and easy — but also by teaching parents how to do specific exercises and stretches with the neck, to help improve range of motion at home. They are gentle exercises as well. Most babies with torticollis are uncomfortable when adjusted, because they don't like to be moved into the restricted positions.

As parents and doctors, we need to encourage the child during the motion exercises, letting them know that everything is okay, rewarding them through that adjustment, rewarding them through the exercises. A chiropractor will be able to teach parents to do work at home to help maintain the range of motion through childhood.

Caught early enough, it can be resolved quickly, to keep any long-term issues at bay.

If you bring the child in after they have been presenting with torticollis for a while, it may take longer to treat than earlier intervention. I've treated children with severe cases of torticollis, and it does take more time.

As you progress, the child will notice the changes, too. I put children in front of a mirror to assess progress. At first, the child will only be able to turn her head one way. After a while, it is a great experience to watch a child turn her head and see herself on both sides in the mirror. That's kind of fun.

Sometimes I place a parent on either side of the baby, and watch the child actually look and see parents on both sides. It opens up the baby's world, and it's so much fun to see them get excited.

Babies with restricted motion can't respond to sounds normally because they can't turn their heads around in both directions. They must turn their whole body around to see what's making noise. When they regain full range of motion, it is a joy to see them turn in response to a voice.

## Ask Your Chiropractor About Other Symptoms

A chiropractor can help infants and children with other symptoms and conditions in addition to the ones presented here. Some examples are:

- Colic
- Potty-training issues
- Bedwetting issues
- Attention-deficit issues
- Learning problems

There are many others. Understand that you just have to ask.

Whatever your child's challenges are, go to a chiropractor and find out how they can help.

*Chapter* **FIVE**

# Your Chiropractor Can Be a Great Resource

## NUTRITION

With regard to nutrition, there are *diets*, and then there are *ways of life*. A good meal plan, food plan, or way of eating for you is a good fit for your whole family. Create a healthy way of life for your children by creating a healthy way of life for yourself and your family.

Very simply, kids will eat what you eat.

If you are having body dysmorphic problems — obsessing over body flaws — then they're going to grow into having those problems. If you don't eat your vegetables, they're not going to eat vegetables. Healthy eating for the whole family is a wonderful gift you can give your children.

**Proper Diet for Kids and Families**

Here are some guidelines for children as well as adults:

- Make sure every meal contains some protein.

- Beware the carbohydrate-rich filler foods. When you fill kids up with these foods, it's hard to get them to eat protein.

- Children should drink water before every meal once they're old enough.

- Make sure your family's overall diet contains an adequate supply of healthy fats. These healthy fats will keep kids fuller longer and keep their brains working properly.

- Focus on proper nutrition.

- Make sure that everyone eats lots of vegetables and fruits.

- You should be eating twice as many vegetables as fruits. So for every fruit, you must have two servings of vegetables.

- Make sure that everyone has enough calories in their meals to keep them sustained.

- Stay hydrated through the day.

## Over-Snackers

This is a big problem. Again, kids fall into habits that we create for them. The full-grown adults of our society have a tendency to be overweight. We get bored, and we eat. We get emotional, and we eat. We're sad, and we eat. We're at the grocery store, and we eat.

Adults have so many triggers that cause us to overeat, but if you look at your children, you might find that you're creating triggers for them also.

Think about these questions:

When your children are upset in the back of the car, do you give them food?

When your children are bored when you're shopping, do you give them food?

When you want them to be quiet, do you give them food?

Do you give them food when they sit in front of the TV?

If you have all these triggers yourself, it is likely that you are basically training kids to eat in the same way. You have to re-train yourself so you don't continue the cycle:

- When your children say they're bored, don't give them food. Give them water and redirect them.

- Make it your policy that they eat at the kitchen table.

- Don't give children food in the car. They can wait. Besides being an inappropriate snack time meant only to appease boredom and maintain quiet, it is a choking hazard.

- Don't give snacks when children are upset about something, to bribe children, or to appease a bad attitude or you will be turning them into emotional eaters.

- Don't give snacks close to mealtime to tide them over; teach kids it is okay to wait.

- Fill them up with healthy fats and proteins at mealtime, including breakfast.

- Make snacks purposeful, not on-demand or in response to a lapse in activity.

- Time snacks to be a reasonable amount of time between meals. Remember, when babies are nursing, they go two or three hours between meals. If given a good breakfast, a toddler should be able to last at least as long between breakfast and snack.

- Don't allow your toddler to walk around with snack cups, juice boxes, and milk.

- If a child is truly hungry and it is mealtime, set a place at the table.

- At feeding times, stress proper nutrition by offering balanced meals with adequate quantities of vegetables, proteins, and fats. When proper meals are finished, children should be satiated and ready to play actively.

Constant snacking makes children lazy, dependent, and focused on their next snack instead of activity. It is a recipe for creating a teenager and adult with eating problems and obesity. I recognize that over-snacking is something that you may already do, and this may be a difficult transition. Sometimes you need to tough it out to show your kids who is in charge. It will be rewarding for you and your children in the end.

**Picky Eaters**

*Note: Recognizing the difference between picky eaters and those with sensory processing issues is important. We are not discussing sensory issues in this book.*

Having picky eaters could be a whole book in itself. In some cases, you need to teach your kids who's in charge, and if you continue to feed into their every whim, you're doing them a disservice.

My children do not love fish. That is just the way it is. My husband and I eat fish once a week. I do not force my children to have fish once a week, but they have to have it twice a month. Twice a month they have to have it; two bites or three bites. They see it every week, they know it's coming, and they complain about it. They can either eat it or not eat it, but it's going to show up on the next plate if they don't eat it.

For picky eaters, it is important to present choices, but to carefully select the choices you give them. Make it fun, but don't let them set the standards.

If given the option of chicken nuggets, pizza, hot dogs, or macaroni and cheese over broccoli, salmon, or grilled chicken, what do you think they're going to pick?

If given the option between jelly beans and peas, I'm going to pick jelly beans every day.

You need to train your kids. You should not be a short-order cook, serving the whims of your children. Teach them young to eat like the adults eat. Smaller portions, smaller sizes, but they should be able to eat what you eat.

You need to make sure that both you and your children understand who's in control of the food decisions. The children need to understand that the parents are in charge, and the parents need to take that responsibility seriously. Learn to select foods that are part of a healthy family diet.

When you're shopping for food, *don't buy foods that you don't want your children to eat!* That policy will save you a lot of trouble.

Make sure that other parents and guardians are on board and understand what you expect. If you have other childcare providers make sure they know what is expected at meal and snack times.

One other side note:

When you have a very young child with allergies or sensitivities, no matter how hard it is, don't torture that poor child by serving them something else while the family eats pizza.

They're not going to understand, so maybe everyone needs to be gluten free for a while.

Maybe your home needs to be a safe haven where they can go into the pantry and eat whatever is safe for them.

I have too many patients that create a shelf for their allergic child and then tell their child to eat only from that shelf.

How does one child have just a shelf, while your two other kids can go and eat anything?

While your child is little, how about making your house safe for everyone instead?

## NATURAL REMEDIES

Your chiropractor is likely to be a great resource for natural remedies, so be sure to ask questions when you go for a session. A lot of great chiropractors either will have information for you or at least can direct you to the right place to find it.

### Healing Foods

This, topic, again, could be a book on its own. Recognize that the food you put in your body can be truly seen as medicine. Here are just a few facts that you might find interesting:

- If you have pain, you can eat foods that reduce inflammation.

- If you are sick, you can eat foods that can help fight that illness.

- Sugars, gluten, dairy, and other foods can have powerful negative effects on your health.

- Garlic is a natural antibiotic.

- Cinnamon is a natural anti-inflammatory.

There are so many great foods that you can eat to improve your health from the inside, but there are also many foods that you eat that could be making you less healthy. Have that conversation with your provider. Discussing natural remedy foods with your chiropractor or natural healthcare provider can help you understand what to eat and what not to eat in order to feel your best.

Here are some healing foods I always keep in my pantry:

- Garlic
- Cinnamon
- Pineapple
- Oregano
- Onions
- Apple cider vinegar
- Honey

Always keep fresh garlic in your home. Fresh garlic is a natural antibiotic, which can be used for ear infections. It can also be used to help with athlete's foot, or even when you have a bacterial infection. Eating garlic can help in so many ways.

Cinnamon is good for blood pressure issues, or blood conditions, to reduce inflammation.

Pineapple is a natural anti-inflammatory as well. I buy a whole pineapple, instead of buying chunks. Buy the whole pineapple, save the core in the freezer, and when someone has pain add a little bit of that core from the pineapple to a smoothie.

Oregano oil is good for viral and fungal issues.

Onions are number one when there's sickness going around in your house. Slice up onions and put them in a bowl or a jar in the room; they help absorb the germs in the air.

Apple cider vinegar is wonderful for so many ailments. Just one dose of it can help relieve heartburn or acid reflux.

Local raw honey can help with seasonal allergies.

These are just a few examples. See your chiropractor or other health professional and ask for more information on nutrition and healing foods.

## A Note About Sugar

There are many foods that can be utilized to make you feel better, but also recognize there are foods that keep you feeling bad. Sugar is one of them.

Why?

- Sugar creates inflammation in the gut.
- Sugar feeds bacteria.
- Sugar feeds yeast.

When you are sick, you want to cut out as much of the sugar in your diet as possible so that your body can get rid of the microbes you've been feeding. Then you can continue recovering from yeast infections, thrush, or constipation. Sugar is the enemy.

**Essential Oils**

This again could be a whole book. The purpose of this section is not to educate you on *all* essential oils, but to give you a little information on the healing benefits of essential oils.

Essential oils are really the very first forms of medicine in history. If you are interested in obtaining these items, realize that there are good essential oils and there are essential oils that are ineffective. Wonderfully high potency essential oils contain healing properties, and super diluted essential oils only give you a pretty smell.

There are lots of wonderful companies, but you need to understand the differences in quality between oils. Recognize that essential oils can work on healing from the inside and out; not just by smelling them, but using them in various forms.

Lavender is great for calming.

Eucalyptus is great for sinus and congestion.

Arnica oil is great for muscle relief, bruising, and pain.

There are many essential oils available, but rarely can high-quality essential oils be purchased off a shelf in a store. Ask questions. Talk to your chiropractor or your natural healthcare provider about what oils to look for and how to use them.

## Supplements

I often recommend supplements to patients and we carry them in my office. We carry supplements for a wide variety of uses.

There are plenty of companies that make wonderful supplements; however, not all supplements are created equal. There are some out there that say wonderful things on the bottle, but when you look at the ingredients they're actually full of fillers and rubbish and are not good for any purpose. Read the labels carefully.

If your chiropractor provides supplements, it's important to talk about what they have, why they have it, and what would be best, whether it's probiotics or multivitamins.

Make sure that you're not giving your child multivitamins full of sugar, food dyes, and other fillers. Make sure your supplements are always made from whole food and not synthetically formulated vitamins and minerals.

Also, avoid purchasing supplements in warehouses or in mega bottles, because supplements have expiration dates. You don't know how long a bottle has been sitting on a warehouse shelf.

Be careful about purchasing supplements online. When you buy from a third party store, you don't know what you are buying. They could be old, expired products that have had the expiration date washed off to resell.

There are many great doctor-grade supplements that are being illegally sold via Amazon. Amazon cuts them off when they find out. These online companies are not affiliated with the supplement manufacturers and cannot provide support if something goes wrong. I have encountered this reality directly.

Go directly to the brand-name company first and find out where their products are sold. Some companies sell directly through Amazon, increasing reliable safety. Direct sale also demonstrates that the company is going to support their product.

I always tell my patients that it's important to act with due diligence when purchasing supplements outside of your doctor's office.

To summarize:

- Avoid buying supplements in mega stores because you don't know how long they've been sitting on the shelf.

- Check expiration dates.

- Be wary of ordering supplements online if you don't know the original source. Don't buy from a third party.

- Consult with your doctor to find the right supplements for you and your family.

- Make sure your supplements are whole food and not synthetic.

- Read the labels.

- Many chiropractors and natural healthcare providers can give you well-informed recommendations and may carry the supplement that is right for your needs.

As a final note, recognize that while natural remedies, essential oils, and supplements are great options, some may not work for everybody. Some people might be allergic to certain foods or supplements or essential oils. Work with your doctor, your chiropractor, or your natural healthcare provider to find the best products and methods before you go rogue and try to figure it all by yourself.

Make sure you understand how remedies work in conjunction with each other. Talk to your chiropractor or your healthcare provider to find the best formula for you and your family.

Many patients find information on their own using the Internet, which can be problematic. Natural remedies can have powerful effects, and you want to make sure you are using the right ones, prepared properly, and at the right dosages.

Some questions are to ask your health professional:

- Is this natural remedy appropriate for me?
- What is the right dosage?
- Does it interact with other medication?
- Is it safe for children?
- Is the dosage different for children?
- Is it safe for pregnant women?

Talk to your health provider to get the answers to these important questions.

## HEALTH AND WELLNESS

Health and wellness are family affairs. It is best to make sure your family knows why you are doing what you are doing, bringing everyone to the same page. Remember to talk to kids about health issues, but *you*, as the parent, are ultimately in charge of health decisions for your family.

### Fitness

I'm a firm believer in the whole family being active and doing things that are fun together. My kids have to have one extracurricular activity that keeps them active — without performance pressure, though. No pressure. We've done T-ball, soccer, gymnastics, and right now they're taking hip-hop. They love it, they're moving, they're active, and it's social. When my husband and I go to the gym, we do not call it *working out*. We do not work out in our family. We go *get awesome* instead.

"Where is Daddy?"

"He went to get awesome."

"What are you doing, Mom?"

"I'm going to be awesome."

When we talk about it, instead of talking about *work*, we talk about being awesome. That was a major change in how I saw working out and physical activity. It made a change in my own mentality. Now, with my kids, when we go for a walk or we go do things, every time we tell them we're going to get awesome.

So now I hear, "Mom, let's go be awesome together."

If we're going to go hiking?

"How awesome!"

We constantly reiterate this idea and it's so much fun. We do a lot of hiking in my family. Obviously, hiking is not for everybody, but that's something that we like to do together. We have adventures. We try to always keep things awesome. That's been a great blessing for us, changing the way we view exercise. I don't love working out, but I sure love to feel awesome.

If you're a busy mom or you're a stay-at-home mom, move with your kids. Get awesome with your kids. Find ways to get them involved.

Most kids want to do what Mom and Dad are doing. We taught my son at three years old, how to do a proper pushup. Nothing's worth doing if you're not doing it right. Then he loved to show off his pushups. We have a pull-up bar. He can't do pull-ups on his own—he's just seven years old—but we hold him, and he loves to do them.

He says, "Oh, that was awesome, I got three!"

It's always about being awesome. Not work, it's being awesome. Family fitness in our house is about everyone being awesome. Try it!

## Other Doctor Referrals

I work regularly with a lot of doctors to whom I would gladly refer a patient: medical doctors, obstetricians and gynecologists, midwives, holistic dentists, eye doctors, and others. I generally refer to doctors who, in turn, refer to chiropractors.

If you believe in chiropractic for your family, wouldn't you also want to see other doctors who believe in a natural way of healthcare?

For example, I would not refer a patient to an obstetrician who doesn't believe in chiropractic. If my patient has back pain and doesn't want drugs, she needs her doctor to support her choices.

If you are looking for a referral, talk to your chiropractor about who they see, and who they recommend. Ask them about pediatricians, eye doctors, or even veterinarians. Chiropractors are a great resource to talk to about other health professionals who have a natural-minded philosophy of healthcare. Don't just guess. We can help.

## Whole-Family Wellness Programs

A whole-family wellness program is a method by which we, as chiropractors, can help you and your entire family to be healthy and get on the right track for continued wellness.

We want the whole family to be supported. Dad needs his adjustments, and Mom needs hers, and so do the kids. The family needs to keep getting awesome. We want to make sure everybody's eating right and feeling good.

Just because we see the children doesn't mean we can't see the parents. We can talk about *everybody's* health and well-being if we focus on the whole family in a wellness program.

A lot of chiropractors have programs for families like we do. Ask about family wellness programs when you meet with your health professional, or when you're seeking a chiropractor. It's truly a wonderful way to look at healthcare.

Understanding and supporting the needs of a whole family creates better care for everyone. No one should be left out. It's about prevention. It's about staying well. It's about making sure that everybody feels awesome.

# *Conclusion*

In writing this book, I wanted to give you a brief understanding of chiropractic, and why it's important for *everyone*, from birth to death, in daily life. After reading this book, it is my hope that you now have some useful knowledge that you can keep and use, and that you better understand how to take care of yourself and your family.

I want you to be able to make informed decisions when it comes to the health and wellness of your family. If you have the resources to gather the information that you need to answer your questions, then you can make better decisions.

You shouldn't ever blindly follow somebody else. This book may not give the answers that you want to hear. But I hope that it leaves you with a sense of the importance of asking questions and getting answers before you act.

I hope that, after finishing this book, you've gained some information about chiropractic, but more importantly, you have been encouraged to ask more questions. Find a chiropractor to talk to. Talk to somebody in a natural healthcare profession to help you understand and make informed decisions when it comes to healthcare and your family.

Whether you choose to see a chiropractor or not, the Internet is not always the best source for information. Sometimes you must seek professional help or professional care. The Internet does not have all the answers, and quite often can have contradicting answers.

Take the step to find a health professional to talk to and bounce questions off. Seek a doctor who is not going to judge your decisions, but will work with you to come up with the best health plan for you and your family.

You can contact me via my website or business Facebook page — see the next page for contact information — and I will happily answer your questions as best I can, as quickly as I can, no matter where you are.

I encourage you to visit the ICPA website to find a chiropractor in your city, or read articles on issues that interest you. We have a plethora of information on our website, and my husband (who is also a Chiropractor and Functional Medicine Doctor) and I regularly post articles on our Facebook page.

Make informed decisions about your family's health. The only way to do this is to ask questions.

If you don't ask the questions, you're not going to get the answers.

# *Next Steps*

Be sure to visit our website www.HuntforWellness. com.

Like us on Facebook at "Hunt for Wellness."

Find us on Instagram at Hunt4Wellness.

We are local to the Charlotte, North Carolina, area:

Hunt for Wellness/Chiropractic

9422 South Tryon Street

Charlotte, NC 28273

Let Hunt for Wellness be your guide for natural health.

Give our office a call for an appointment today: 704-588-1792

# About the Author

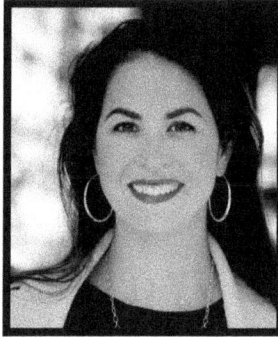

*Estela Hunt, DC*

Dr. Estela is a native of Florida where she attended high school in Miami and Rollins College in Winter Park. After graduating from Rollins College, she became a licensed massage therapist where she crafted her skill of muscle work and enjoyed working for the Disney resorts. Her ultimate goal, however, was to become a chiropractor and she eventually moved to St. Louis, Missouri, where she attended Logan College of Chiropractic.

Dr. Estela's desire to become a chiropractor was one that stemmed from her own personal experience as a teenager. After suffering from excruciating leg and hip pain with running or walking, her parents took her to a chiropractor. Dr. Estela saw first-hand the power of the chiropractic adjustment; not only did her leg and hip pain disappear, but she joined the cross-country track team.

Dr. Estela has a passion to help all people but her specialty is children. As a mother of two, she knows the importance of having healthy kids. She has dedicated the last few years to extensive training in the care of pediatrics and prenatal chiropractic.

When asked to summarize her vision, she states, "There is nothing more rewarding than parents who exclaim how thankful they are when their children are no longer suffering from being colicky, irritable, or sick. Then, they and their children can finally rest."

www.ingramcontent.com/pod-product-compliance
Lightning Source LLC
Chambersburg PA
CBHW052222270326
41931CB00011B/2448

* 9 7 8 1 9 4 5 4 4 6 1 3 9 *